BECOMING A

NURSING ASSISTANT

Enjoy The Extensive Rewards Of A Nursing Assistant Career

Copyright 2009

KMS Publishing.com

With so many possible careers to choose from, why should one choose to become a Nurse Assistant?

While some people view the Nurse Assistant as lower level staff in the medical profession, it actually takes an extraordinary individual to take on a Nursing Assistant position. Any person can use intellect and go through training and education, but it demands amazing skills of compassion, dedication, patience, a genuine sincerity to help others, and excellent communication skills to relate with different personalities day in and day out to accomplish tedious tasks.

It can be a very rewarding occupation that offers high pay and the highly coveted chance to work with people and to work in the prestigious medical field. The career is in very high demand nowadays, so employment choices are numerous.

So, how can you launch your career as a Nursing Assistant? This manual can help show you how. We present information on what the CNA role demands from you so that you get into the job fully-prepared. Obtain valuable information on education, training, and licensing so you get the full benefit of the job. We give you career options and guidelines for career development and advancement so you can continue to be the best in your field even if a new generation of Nursing Assistants endangers your position.

Learn the real secrets of successful Nursing Assistants so you can become one of them!

TABLE OF CONTENTS

INTRODUCTION

Becoming a nursing assistant is really a calling to many individuals. It takes a special person and a specific type of personality to be attracted to the nursing assistant profession. You are a huge part of patient care and for many people that can be a draw, though it does have its challenges. You are there to assist your patients with their most basic and fundamental needs, and you are the right hand to the nursing staff at your chosen medical facility. You need to know what it takes to be compassionate, patient, helpful, and discreet as you will help patients with needs that they are used to handling on their own.

To get the call and decide that a profession as a nursing assistant is an excellent first step—and an important one at that! For some, a career as a nursing assistant is a final destination and one in which they center their working life around. However there are many individuals who chose to become a nursing assistant on their road to becoming a registered nurse. Perhaps they are not ready to travel the long road to a role as a registered nurse or they are at a point in their life where they need to start working as they pursue the schooling. Nursing school can not only be a huge financial burden, but also a rather large commitment taking time away from other aspects of the life. Whatever your chosen path is as you enter into the world of the nursing assistant role, know that what you are getting into can be extremely rewarding and at times rather demanding as well.

Most individuals who pursue a career as a nursing assistant will need to become a Certified Nursing Assistant (CNA) as this is highly desirable. It can be possible to become a nursing assistant without education in certain facilities, but the majority of them require that an individual be a CNA to be hired. This can mean longevity and a more desirable salary, and is definitely a requirement for those who wish to pursue a more involved nursing profession. Whether you chose to make your long-term career goals as a nursing assistant or it is a stop along the way towards becoming a registered nurse, it's important to understand the role, responsibilities, and requirements for a CNA.

Being a nursing assistant can bring great satisfaction to an individual's life and can provide great comfort to those around you. You will be depended on by the nursing staff for which you serve, as well as the patients which you care for. You can find great fulfillment through your commitment and your tasks in patient care and can learn some excellent lifelong skills in the process. Within the chapters of this book we will look at what it takes to be an excellent nursing assistant, what the expectations and responsibilities are, how you can go about becoming a CNA, and finally what such a profession can mean in your life.

1

THE JOB DESCRIPTION OF A NURSING ASSISTANT

Most people hear of the profession of a nursing assistant and are unsure of what exactly that means or just how much it entails. The nursing assistant can often be considered the "unsung hero" as they are in the background performing many of the responsibilities that patients or their families may take for granted. It is quite common that nursing assistants pay special care to the fundamental and daily needs of a patient so that the nurse can focus on some of the more involved procedures and tasks. Oftentimes a registered nurse is the only one capable of performing certain responsibilities by law, and therefore must rely on their nursing assistant to help with daily tasks.

A nursing assistant helps with many of the needs that a patient may have, some of which are not always easy or desirable. It takes a patient and compassionate person to be able to properly handle the tasks associated with patient care. Nursing assistants can be expected to help with doing everything from answering patient's calls to their room to helping them to build up their physical activity. As you can expect to find nursing assistants in any type of medical facility from hospitals to nursing homes, the responsibilities will certainly vary based on the type of patient and their associated needs.

Emergency Response

As with any other type of medical professional, it's important that a nursing assistant be well versed in emergency care. There will be the instance throughout the career of a nursing assistant in which they may very well be faced with an emergency type of situation and they must know what to do and be clear on how to properly proceed. This is important to keep the patient calm and to properly diagnose and deal with the situation at hand. It's safe to say then that a nursing assistant must be able to keep calm and handle stress properly when these types of situations arise. Without a clear head, a nursing assistant can only add to an already stressful situation so being calm, cool, and collected in times of trauma can be of great help. This is worth considering when one begins down the path towards a nursing assistant.

Compassionate Aid

It's also important to know that a nursing assistant may have to deal with some difficult situations that require dignity and compassion. One such situation that may arise is when a nursing assistant is working with the elderly or bed ridden patient for whom they must assist with simple but important personal and private care. Patients will often require a bed pan and assistance with collecting urine or feces so it's important to remember this as it will be a part of a nursing assistant career. Patients rely on nursing assistants for their daily care and it's important to remember that they are at the mercy of those who care for them.

Accurate Care

A nursing assistant may be required to keep a close eye on the intake of a patient for a variety of medical reasons. There are many medical reasons which may dictate a patient be observed in their food and liquid consumption, and oftentimes a nursing assistant is the one who oversees such activity. Therefore it's important that a nursing assistant be observant, diligent, detail oriented and accurate as they handle and oversee such an important and precise type of activity.

In most instances, a nursing assistant is not the one who administers medication. By law, it must be the registered nurse who handles such a need for the patient but they will often work hand in hand with the nursing assistant to ensure that the intake is in line with the needs for the medication to be administered. You can quickly see how the nursing assistant forms the basis for the medical team which cares for each and every patient that walks through the doors of the given medical facility. It's important to have the type of personality who can blend well with an often stretched nursing staff and for whom can handle the most private of patients needs.

The C.N.A. As An Avenue To The Nursing World

Nursing assistants wear many hats and often have to work with many different types of personalities so this is an important consideration as one begins their path towards this type of career. It's also important to remember that if one wishes to pursue a career as a registered nurse later on that they observe as much as possible. As one works in a career as a CNA, they can usually learn a lot from the registered nurses around them. Taking this on as a learning phase and asking questions can only make for a better candidate later on. It's always a good idea to be sure that a career as a registered nurse is a good match and there's no better way to evaluate such a thing as to work side by side with them. Each type of nurse has their own sets of responsibilities that come along with it. A nursing assistant is an excellent way to dip your foot in the water of the nursing world and to evaluate what it's all about and if it is in fact a match for you.

Those patients that require the most attention can be challenging at times, but often provide the greatest rewards. As a nursing assistant you can fully expect that you will have to care for patients who are bed ridden, incapable of walking or moving, or who are physically or mentally impaired. For some, this may be just why they pursue a career as a nursing assistant so that they may care for those with special needs. You may have to help move such an individual, feed them, or just provide general care. For some people this may be tough as you are the source of their every need, but for others this type of patient can prove to be the most rewarding. Being able to provide the most basic and involved care can help to remind many of what a career as a nursing assistant is all about and why so many feel so passionate about it and their role in helping others.

Your Stepping Stone To A Nursing Career

A Nursing Assistant certificate allows you the opportunity to secure employment at entry level in the medical field. This position requires compassion and dedication to assisting others. It also requires a high level of effective communication as well as attention for detail. Most people entering the Nursing Assistant profession find it to be a rewarding and challenging career. However, many choose to use it as a building block for becoming a Nurse.

The program for becoming a Nursing Assistant is very fast compared with the time it takes to earn a degree in Nursing. Therefore, many see it as a logic choice to gain experience in the medical field. It is an excellent idea for those that aren't sure if Nursing is for them. It is better to spend four to twelve weeks in training to find out then to spend two or more years working on a Nursing degree.

There are individuals who must maintain employment while pursuing their education degree for financial reasons. For individuals in this position, completing the Nursing Assistant program offers them a way to secure employment that is related to what they are going to school for.

Others choose to advance their career once they have been working as a Nurse Assistant because they see many of the tasks Nurses are responsible for. It is a level of responsibility they wish to acquire. Since they work so closely with the Nursing staff, it is a perfect opportunity to explore more of what takes place. Others have a sincere desire to further their education, but for a variety of reasons have not been able to.

There is a significant pay difference between working as a Nursing Assistant and having a degree as a Nurse. The dollar amount varies based on location, but on average the difference is $4 to $9 per hour more. It doesn't take long at all for the overall income difference to be seen. Nursing assistants often decide that they want to work in the medical field, but definitely want to be paid more for their work. Of course, the level of responsibility differs greatly between a Nursing Assistant and a Nurse.

Working at a medical facility as a Nursing Assistant can work to your advantage when you decide to pursue a degree in Nursing. It might help you get into the program if there is more interest in the program than enrollment opportunities.

Due to the continuous demand for qualified trained professionals in the area of Nursing, most medical facilities will support you in your efforts to further your education.

They will often adjust your work schedule to accommodate you whenever possible.

Tuition assistance programs are offered by many employers in the medical field. They work in a variety of ways. Some will cover a percentage of your tuition; others will pay up to a particular dollar amount. Often, you will be required to agree to work for them for a particular length of time or have to reimburse them for any tuition paid on your behalf. Others won't pay anything while you are attending school, but will offer tuition reimbursement upon completion of your Nursing degree.

Another advantage of working as a Nursing Assistant prior to obtaining your degree in Nursing is you will have an edge over other recent graduates. You will have work experience to offer in combination with your degree while many others will only have their degree.

Employers like to maintain their quality employees. If you are able to show outstanding work ethic as a Nursing Assistance, it is very likely they will offer you a position as a Nurse upon your completion of your degree. This often depends on the job openings at the medical facility you work for.

Your certificate and work experience as a Nurse Assistant can help make career opportunities appear. It may peak your interest in returning to school to work on your Nursing degree for a variety of reasons. It can help you be accepted to a Nursing program, as well as help you secure employment after completing your Nursing degree.

A Typical Day For The Nursing Assistant

It's important to keep in mind that as a nursing assistant you are often involved with extensive periods of standing or being on your feet, as well as lifting heavy loads. Having the ability to lift or move patients either within their bed or from one surface to another can be a heavy burden for some. It's important to remember that these patients depend on the nursing assistants that care for them and they are at their mercy. The patients and their families put their trust into your hands as a nursing assistant and therefore you must be able to offer all of the characteristics that you would want out of somebody caring for your very own loved one.

While there is no one typical day when it comes to the life of a nursing assistant, there are certain responsibilities that are quite common. These include:

- Answering patient's call lights to assist with needs as they come up

- Serving patients meals and in some cases actually feeding them

- Transporting patients between locations throughout the medical facility or outside points

- Lifting patients or turning them within their bed

- Keeping patients dry, helping to change soiled linens or gowns as necessary

- Collecting any required specimens such as urine or feces

- Observing and noting patient's daily habits, food or liquid consumption, or behavioral patterns

- Assisting the nursing staff on any required tasks involving patient care

- Keeping the line of communication open with the patient and their family

- Performing any necessary grooming that the patient may require

- Washing clothes and linens for the patients each day

- Ensuring that all of patient care provided is of the utmost quality

Obviously the amount of work involved and care required is dependent on the needs of the patients that a nursing assistant has in her facility. It can be helpful to consider what types of special responsibilities may be involved with the medical facilities that you may work for as a nursing assistant. Patient care is the number one priority no matter where you work as a nursing assistant and understanding that is an excellent start.

Confidentiality Equals Professionalism

Nursing Assistants are exposed to a wide variety of events taking place in the medical field. It is crucial that they are aware of the importance of maintaining confidentiality in all aspects of their job.

Nursing Assistants are well trained in the policies and procedures of the facility. While it is important to follow them, it is not recommended to discuss them outside of the facility. For example, you don't want to provide others with confidential information regarding evacuation and other emergency procedures. Doing so many compromise the safety of the patients and staff during a natural disaster or violent attack.

Patients requiring care in a medical facility are to have their privacy protected. This means you do not discuss their care or other personal information with any other person except staff they have an interest in the care of that patient. Confidentiality becomes an issue when you know someone in the facility or someone asks you why someone else in there.

All patients have the right to their privacy being maintained. Compromising this information is a direct violation of every medical practice. Providing such information can result in termination of your job, and in some cases, the loss of your Nursing Assistant Certification.

Communicable diseases can surface in medical facilities. It is important that you follow the policies and procedures set in place by the particular facility your work with. However, do not release information regarding such diseases to anyone. This could result in a panic over the possibility of an epidemic, and lead to patients wanting to leave the facility against medical advice.

The proper medical staff will release information on communicable diseases to the proper agencies. Often this includes the area health department. They can then help the medical facility incorporate a plan of action to remedy the solution. The decision might be made to share the information with the area newspapers in an effort to allow them to protect themselves and to seek medical attention if they display the symptoms of a communicable disease that requires treatment.

Confidentiality also includes other medical staff. Nursing Assistants should not be disclosing any information they overhear among other staff in regards to a patient. Likewise, they should not disclose any information that they hear about the private interactions of staff. Often referred to as gossip, this violation of confidentiality can result in poor working relationships. The result is often a stressful work environment and patients not receiving the best care because lines of communication are not open.

To protect yourself, it is important that you clearly understand the basics of confidentiality and why it is so important in the Nursing Assistant profession. Make sure you are fully aware of the specific policies and procedures in place for the facility you work for prior to accepting employment. In addition, it is the responsibility of the Nursing Assistant to report any violations of the confidentiality policies and procedures to the proper person. Not doing so makes you as much a part of the violation as those who committed it.

While it is human nature to talk and discuss things in common, make sure the information you are sharing in regards to your work are being shared with those who need to know the information. It can be humiliating enough for individuals who need to be in a medical facility without worrying about who is going to find out about what took place while they were in care.

2

THE CNA PROGRAM REQUIREMENTS

There are ways to launch into the nursing profession without obtaining a certification, but it's rather limited. A nurse's aide doesn't require any training but there is limited capacity for what this role may do and the salary is also at a bare minimum as well. When it comes to becoming a nursing assistant, the best route to take is to obtain a certification and become a full-fledged Certified Nursing Assistant (CNA). The requirements are certainly not as stringent as those for becoming a registered nurse or for getting a degree, but there are a certain number of hours involved in training in the classroom as well as working in a medical facility.

Certification

To become a CNA, requires a certification of at least 75 hours in basic healthcare, medical ethics, and health law. The specific requirements vary by state but it's essential that to become a CNA, an individual must have a common and inherent knowledge of medical practices and how healthcare works. As you consider this education, you want to search for a program that fits your specific needs. There are a number of different program types available that can cater to your individual lifestyle, budgetary or time constraints, or that can take you on the fast track and get you through the program quickly and efficiently. The choice is yours!

Consider Lifestyle Commitments

First and foremost, you want to consider your lifestyle and current commitments. There are some CNA programs that run all day as a full time commitment each week. While others are offered only as night classes to accommodate those that are already working and need to allot time for classes around their already busy schedules. You can even find some programs that are offered strictly and wholly online to work around your schedule. For example if you have children that you are trying to work around, you could find a program that fits into your busy schedule and allows you to still be home when your kids are. There is a program for everybody making it seamless to log in the required hours to obtain your CNA certification.

The good news is that there are so many resources online to help you in your search for the perfect CNA program. You can find programs through local universities, online resources, or through medical facilities directly. In this day and age, finding a program that works best for you is much easier than it ever used to be. As you begin your search it can be helpful to remember what sorts of requirements your specific state has. Take the time to research what you will need to do, the hours that you will need to log, and what options you have available to fill all of the necessary requirements. Then you can base your schedule around the requirements to be sure to zero in on the program that works best for you.

The CNA Program Selection Criteria

As you look into a wide array of different CNA programs, consider the criteria that are most important to you. Look at various factors such as:

- What other commitments do you currently have?

- What time of day would classes be most convenient for you?

- Are you disciplined enough and equipped to handle all online classes?

- Is your lifestyle conducive to being in class each day of the week?

- Is there a convenient location for you to take classes near home?

- How quickly do you want to get your CNA certification?

- Is money a factor in taking classes? Is there any financial help available?

- Do you work best in a classroom setting with others or working independently?

As with any educational program, there is a good fit for everyone. There are certain personalities that do well with a traditional classroom type of setting, while others do much better working on their own. If you choose something like online classes, be aware that you must have a great discipline to turn away other distractions and focus on your work. Think through every aspect of the curriculum and program that you are looking at and be sure that it fits your life and everything you have going on within it.

Finding a CNA program that works best for you and fits your needs is the first and most important step towards your success. If you start such a program on the right foot, it will be a great way to secure your success and longevity in the future. Be honest with yourself about what you can accommodate with your current lifestyle as rushing through a program or trying to squeeze it in can really hurt you later. Take the time and clear your calendar as much as possible to ensure that the program you select will provide you with the solid foundation that you need to be successful in your future as a nursing assistant. This is the first step towards a very important decision in your life, so be sure to make it last and allow yourself to search around and find the program that is best for you.

College Options

Now what you have decided to start looking into a career as a nursing assistant you will want to consider your options for obtaining the education you need to go into your newly chosen field.

There are many options to consider when deciding to go into nursing assisting as a career choice. Many city and state level colleges will offer programs to help you start as a Nursing assistant however one of the more popular methods for obtaining a nursing assistant certification is through a vocational or career training school.

Some of the more popular Nursing training schools are St. Augustine Educational Services which can be found at http://nursingassistant.us, Concorde career colleges which can be found at www.Concorde.edu, and also another very popular school is Bryman college at www.Go2BrymanCollege.com

While you can expect to make good money as a Nursing assistant, some of the schooling to get you started will be an expense that you need to seriously consider and plan for.

During the research that we did when writing this article we found that on average Nursing assistant school vocational colleges ranged between $2500 and $6,000 to give you the certification that you need to get started right away. A few schools have all expenses included however others do have material fees of up to $2500 which will want to be considered when making your choice an educational institution.

A few schools such as American career colleges www.americancareer.info offer not only Nursing assistant educations but also dental assistant, pharmaceutical, x-ray, and nursing educations all under one roof. One of these type schools might be a great choice for you if you're not 100% sure that a career as a Nursing assistant is your final destination. By going to a college or career center that offers multiple medical field positions you will be putting yourself in a great position to see exactly what all of your options are when considering a career in the health industry.

A school such as this also would be a great place to continue your education after receiving your certification a Nursing assistant, to possibly move up to a career as a RN or even possibly continue your education in the future to become a doctor.

Starting now and an industry that is growing as rapidly as the health care industry is in today's world is a great way to insure you will have the skills necessary to maintain an excellent career in the health field.

With the skills you are about to learn as a nursing assistant you'll find jobs are not hard to find if you are skilled and professional at your newfound craft.

There's a great sense of self-satisfaction to be had in knowing that you're doing something that helps other people and improves the quality of life for many.

One area to consider if you like children is to specialize in medical practices that cater specifically to children. Specialized practices like this are a great way to carve yourself into a niche area of the market that is always guaranteed to be highly profitable and busy.

Working with children can be one of the most rewarding parts of a nursing career and I highly recommend it as a specialty area for anyone considering a career in dentistry that also has a fondness of children.

So whether you're deciding to go into nursing assistant career college as just a stepping stone for a career as a

Nurse or doctor, or if working as a Nursing assistant is to be your final destination I want to say congratulations on your choice to look into the Nursing assistant field and may have much success in your endeavors.

3

METHODS FOR CNA CERTIFICATION

Now begins a very exciting time in your life—you are about to begin your very important CNA training program. You've carefully researched all of the programs in your area and found the one that best fits your needs. You have an idea of what to expect, but until you get into the actual certification program, it can all be a bit uncertain. Some will receive their CNA certification through a community college as it's the best resource in terms of the cost—usually anywhere between $1000-5000. Others will receive their certification through an actual medical facility. Still others will do all of their work through online courses. It matters not where you get your CNA certification from, it matters that you've made the leap and you are now going for it.

The Value Of Real World Application

A very popular route that many seem to be choosing for their CNA certification is on-the-job options. These offer money towards your education and the attainment of your required credit hours, while allowing you to gain valuable real world experience. Whether you choose this route or not, it can be advised to get some practical experience either before or as you work towards your CNA certification. This can help you to bring the lessons you will learn in the classroom into the real world and see just how you will handle the situations that arise in the profession.

Working in a medical facility or nursing home while you go for your schooling can also help you to secure a position after you have completed your training requirements. It used to be that many of these facilities were short handed and that they were in desperate need of staff. However times have changed and as a nursing assistant has become one of the fastest growing professions, it can help you so much later on if you get in some experience. This will not only help you to truly master the lessons you are learning in the classroom, but it will allow you to be competitive amongst others going through the same training program that you are.

State Requirements

It's important to note that the requirements for a CNA certification program vary by state. Each state mandates what an individual needs to learn and pass in order to gain their certification; these are regulated by the state governments and are subject to change at any time. It's helpful to know up front what your individual state requires so that you are sure that the program you are enrolled in meets the qualifications, but chances are that you're safe if it's an accredited program.

There are some standardized requirements that seem to be common amongst states, and these include:

- Successfully passing a CNA certification program

- 75 hours of a CNA training course that are logged and recorded

- 16 hours of the course must be supervised in a clinical type of setting for real world type of experience

- A final test must be passed to measure the individual's skills taught and gained in the CNA class

- Mastering of fundamental but essential skills such as CPR, bathing, caring for, and feeding patients

- 12 hours of continuing education taken each year to stay certified in the given state

These are usually the fundamental requirements for an individual to pass before they can gain their CNA certification. Some states have additional requirements or rules that must be followed before the certification is given. Others have more lenient requirements, so it's definitely worth checking into. It can also be beneficial to check into the requirements of other states if you ever plan on getting a job elsewhere. You may have to take additional classes or fulfill other requirements if you were ever to move and plan on being a CNA in another state.

Basic Licensing Requirements

For those interested in pursuing a career in the medical field, obtaining your certification as a Nursing Assistance can be exactly what you are looking for. While the specifications for licensing vary by state, all programs have basic elements. First, you must be able to pass a background check. This is for the safety of all patients and other staff. Some states only look at felony convictions, while others look for reckless behaviors including harassment, domestic violence, and driving under the influence of alcohol. Most programs also require a GED or High School diploma.

Nursing Assistant programs are generally run by healthcare facilities and local colleges. Contact any such facility for a listing of up coming classes in your area. Generally, the courses run from four weeks to twelve weeks in length. You will be required to complete a set amount of hours of classroom time as well as a set amount of hours of clinicals. These clinicals are hands on practice that takes place at a medical facility. You will not be paid for your hours worked during this training program. Federal law requires a minimum of 75 hours in any program, all of which must be supervised by a qualified Registered Nurse.

Upon completing all of your classroom hours and clinical training, you will then be required to take a Certified Nursing Assistant exam. This exam is held periodically throughout each state. Some agencies will allow you to secure employment as a Nursing Assistant during that period of time between completing the program and your scheduled exam. Often, verification of program completion and verification that you are registered to take the test are sufficient.

This comprehensive exam is made up of two parts, written and clinical. The written part of the test is said to be mainly common sense. The clinical portion will require you to perform a number of techniques that you will be using in your job. You Nursing Assistant program instructor will inform you of items you should be well skilled in for the exam. In addition, forming your own study group and taking online practice tests can help you feel confident as the date of the test arrives.

The Nursing Assistant licensing requirements are designed to ensure everyone obtaining a certification from the program is properly trained in policies and procedures. Precautions are taken for the safety of the patients, their families, and other medical staff members. It is important to understand that the program will only help you to learn the basics of the job. The specific job requirements will depend on the facility you are working for. You will receive either orientation or on the job training at each medical facility you begin employment with in the area of Nursing Assistant.

With the demand for Nursing Assistants very high right now, it is an excellent career to pursue. The demand is anticipated to continue growing, with the biggest demands being in facilities caring for the elderly. This is the result of people living longer on average.

If you have any questions about the Nursing Assistant licensing requirements in your state, contact your state Medical Board by phone or online. The interest also provides you will additional information on licensing, classes, and career development in the area of Nursing Assistant.

Curriculum Expectations

You can expect the foundation and bulk of a CNA certification course to be just like any other classroom setting. You will be given a great deal of material on everything related to patient care, fundamental medical information, and anything related to the job and its responsibilities. You will be taught how to properly care for a patient, how to administer CPR, what to do in certain situations, and a wide array of other topics. The training for a nursing assistant varies in length depending on the actual program that you select, but it can take anywhere from a couple of weeks to a couple of months. It's important to truly focus on the subject matter at hand because in this certification program, you are learning all of the ins and outs that will pertain to your daily life on the job. This is an excellent depiction of what it will be like to work as a nursing assistant and the entire curriculum is developed around the first hand perspective.

Many times you may even find that a CNA certification course is actually taught by a real life registered nurse. This can be that much more helpful to the students within the classroom as they can understand how it all works from a firsthand perspective and ask all of the pertinent questions that may come up as they go through the course material. You will be walked through the fundamental duties, how the responsibilities work in a real life setting, and see what a day in the life of a nursing assistant. Consider yourself lucky if the course is taught by a registered nurse as this can be your single best source for showing you the ropes and guiding you through what you can expect.

Take advantage of any of the real life setting scenarios you are faced with in your CNA course. Whether you are learning in the classroom, performing role plays with fellow students in your class, or logging your actual training hours, this is what makes for a true distinction amongst other professions. To be a truly successful nursing assistant, you can find that paying close attention and working well in your real life scenarios can be the best preparation you can ask for.

On The Job Training Focus

You will undoubtedly learn a great deal of useful information in the classroom. You'll be taught many useful skills and understand the basics of fundamental health and medical care. This can come in handy as your profession as a nursing assistant and will teach you lessons that you can likely take with you into other aspects of your life. However as most CNA training course also allow you to have true on the job training, this is where you really want to focus your attention and be sure that all of your questions are answered.

While it may seem easy initially to see what patient care is all about and what it entails, there's a great deal of attention involved with it. The fact that the majority of CNA certification courses give you the opportunity to log actual training hours in the field presents you with a very distinct and helpful training regimen. Take advantage of any patient care that you get to observe or assist with because this experience or vantage point will come in quite handy later on. You may find yourself in a situation where you are trying to lift a patient or move them on the bed they are restricted to and you will find that looking back on your training course can be quite helpful. Even something that sounds simplistic such as gathering specimens, feeding a patient, or tracking the eating habits of a patient can all be made much easier if you get the necessary on the job training.

There are also some very important medical procedures that you will likely be involved with for which your on the job training can be extremely valuable. You will often be asked to measure a patient's vital signs, and though this may sound easy or you think that you have the hang of it, you never know until you are faced with it in real life. Observe as much as you possibly can through the on the job training that you are provided with, it will pay off later on. Measuring a patient's vital signs are part of it but administering CPR can be another big part of the job. It's not to say that every day you will be faced with a situation that warrants CPR or that there won't be others that can help such as a registered nurse. However as you will likely be working in either a medical facility or a nursing home, the need for understanding how to administer CPR can be quite helpful and come in handy later on.

Clinicals

Nurse Assistants play a vital role in our healthcare facilities. They provide patients with assistance in regard to their basic needs including bathing, feeding, and dressing them. The level of assistance depends on the individual needs of each patient. They also are an invaluable resource for the Nursing staff.

Becoming a Nurse Assistant requires completion of a certificate program. Such programs are available at several medical facilities and college campuses. The programs can be completed in as little as four weeks. Others run as long as twelve weeks. It depends on the curriculum, the requirements of the state the program is taking place in, and how many hours per day the course is conducted.

All Nurse Assistance courses will teach you the basic fundamentals of taking care of those under your care in a safe and professional manner. Your work will be supervised by licensed Nurses both during your training and regular employment. The training program will teach you to care for both the physical and psychological needs of each patient. Since you must successfully pass the Certified Nursing Assistant exam, the course will help you prepare for the information on that exam.

During the Nurse Assistant course, you will be involved in learning textbook materials as well as hands on training. The textbook material cover all the terminology and information you need to lay a solid foundation to build on. This information will also cover items that are likely to be found on the Certified Nursing Assistant exam. You will also learn ways to improve your communication skills. Communication is key to being a great Nurse Assistant. You will need to be effective at communicating with patients, their family, and the other medical staff.

The hands on portion of the training will give you the opportunity to practice the concepts you are learning in the classroom. Most training programs have special medical mannequins that you work with. You will practice proper bathing and lifting on them. You may also practice taking their vital signs as some are designed for that purpose.

The majority of Nurse Assistant programs work with in conjunction with the medical facilities in the area. This often means a large portion of your hands on training will take place as such a facility. This portion of the curriculum is called clinicals. During this process, you will tend to real patients with the close supervision of licensed medical staff. You will begin applying your knowledge in this setting.

Clinicals can be intimidating to some students. However, they are designed to give you the best opportunity to fully understand and learn your role as a Nurse Assistant. Generally, these clinicals are conducted with a very small group of students. Your class will be broke up into groups of at least two but no more than six. They take place in the actual medical facility. It is important to understand that you will not be paid for the work you do during these clinical hours of training.

During clinicals, the Nursing staff is fully aware of your inexperience. They will attempt to explain what is taking place as it happens to improve your ability to look for key factors in a medical setting. It is very important that if you do not fully understand something, that you discuss it with those training you. They are there for that purpose during the training portions of the Nurse Assistant program.

Completing your Nurse Assistant training at a medical facility not only gives you hands on experience, it may lead to a job offer at the end of your training program. Many medical facilities that host the clinical training are watching out for students who show potential. They are looking for punctuality, attendance, attention to detail, a willingness to learn, and a positive attitude.

On advantage of accepting a job offer at the facility you completed your clinical training at is that you will know their policies and procedures. It is important to keep in mind that every facility has variations of how you were training. The basics will be the same, but you will need to be willing to adjust to what is expected at the particular facility you accept employment with. Keeping that in mind, you will want to ask questions of that nature during job interviews if a complete job description is not given to you.

The Exam & Ongoing Education

Not only will you get the great on the job training that you will need later on, as well as learn the valuable lessons that the curriculum provides, but you will have to apply all of this to the exam. This is where paying attention really comes in handy—if you ask the right questions and truly absorb the material, then passing the exam at the end will be a breeze! To be a successful nursing assistant and have the necessary CNA certification, you must first pass the exam. This will come at the end of the course and measure your knowledge of all of the important subject matters. This is when it truly pays to not only be a good student, but to be one that is focused on and truly passionate about this new profession before you.

Adding to the likelihood of successfully passing the class is to practice the lessons that you learn. Apply them in the on the job training, use them at home to be sure that you master them and understand them. So much of patient care is about practicing and getting better and more well versed, and you will become more agile and far more likely to pass your exam by practicing the lessons you are taught. You will be measured on everything that you learned and there's a great deal of information thrown at you at once, so take your time to really study up. If you pass then you are officially certified, but if you do not then you have a lot more work to do and will likely have to repeat the course.

For most people, once they get into the real life lessons and see how they will be working, this can seal the deal and provide an excellent motivation to pass the test and be done once and for all. Take your time, ask plenty of questions along the way, and study up so that you are sure to get the passing result you want and move on with your career as a nursing assistant. Once you pass, the pressure is off and you can begin your new and exciting career. Your CNA certification is yours to keep and cherish, you just have to be sure to remember to take any necessary courses to keep your certification going each and every year. Again this will vary by state but the continuing education requirement is usually minimal and in place to ensure that you are keeping current with trends and staying fresh within your profession.

Helpful Tips For Preparing For The CNA Exam

Pursing a certificate as a Nursing Assistant is a very exciting adventure. The curriculum generally lasts from four to twelve weeks depending on the requirements in your state. Federal regulations require a minimum of seventy five hours of training. You Nursing Assistant course will be composed of classroom training, practicing what you learned on mannequins and each other, and clinicals that involve working with actual clients in a medical facility under the supervision of a Registered Nurse.

Upon completing your certification, you will be required to take the Certified Nursing Assistant Exam. Most states require you to sign up for the test within ninety days of completing all course work. Your program is set up to specifically teach you the fundamentals you will need on the job as well as to pass the exam. It is your responsibility to ask for clarification of any areas you are unsure of prior to taking the Nursing Assistant exam.

While the Certified Nursing Assistant Exam requirements will vary from state to state, most are very similar in structure and content. The test is made up of two parts – written and clinical. The written portion of the test will contain questions about basic concepts and procedures. Your course textbooks and class notes are excellent studying resources.

The clinical portion of the exam requires you to demonstrate anywhere from three to five Nursing Assistant skills you should have mastered during your program. You will need to perform these skills for a state examiner who will be watching your every move. These skills involve hand washing, privacy, dignity, providing a bed pan, re-positioning a patient in their bed, grooming, taking a patient's temperature, and completing a linen change with the occupant still in the bed.

While hand washing, privacy, and dignity may all seem like common sense areas to many of us, they are very important. Since most communicable diseases can be eliminated by proper hand washing, this skill is absolutely necessary. Providing all patients with privacy and dignity are the cornerstone of any area of the medical profession.

They are relevant to the many duties of Nursing Assistants.

Most people are very nervous about this portion of the test, but practicing correct processed during your program and on your own will help you be prepared. Forming study groups with classmates is an excellent way to practice for both the written and clinical portions of the test. There are also study guides available and online practice tests.

The state examiner understands that exams are stressful and make people nervous. They will be watching to see how you react under stress and pressure because these skills are also important for Nursing Assistants to acquire.

Passing your Nursing Assistant exam is very important. Some employers will hire you once you have completed the program, but you must provide verification that you also passed your state exam within a specified timeframe to maintain that employment. Most states will allow you to find out right after the exam if you have passed or not. You will have the opportunity to retest if you don't pass the first time. There are rules regarding how many times you can take the test, the length of time between each testing, and the cost to retest. These things all vary by state guidelines.

4

RESPONDING TO THE HIGH DEMAND OF NURSING ASSISTANTS

Here's the good news for those that are about to embark into the world of being a Certified Nursing Assistant (CNA)—this is a position that is in high demand! Even in tough economic times or when there are high unemployment rates, there is usually a need for certain medical professions. The medical community rarely goes into a holding pattern, particularly when times get tough. People will always require good and proper medical attention and they will always need people to nurse them back to health. This becomes especially important when you consider that a nursing assistant is one of the most fundamental and necessary when it comes to good solid patient care.

It used to be that people underestimated the profession of a nursing assistant. When there was a nursing shortage in general, people just assumed that a registered nurse could do it all and find the time to provide key medical procedures as well as handle the often demanding patient care. Times have sure changed! Not only is the medical community understanding and embracing the importance of nursing in general, but they are also seeing just how important each level is to ensure the very best in patient care. Most registered nurses are often overworked and have a great deal of responsibilities to handle for each patient in conjunction with the doctors. That means that the nursing assistant plays a vital role in ensuring that the patient is taken care of, comfortable, and in the state required for their specific health condition.

_Align Your Job Search To Your CNA Career Choice

As with any other job search, you need to have a starting point. You need to step back and take a look at where you really see yourself working. You've already taken the big plunge and decided that a career as a nursing assistant is for you. You've found the right CNA program that matches your needs, and once you've successfully passed your certification exam you want to be able to jump into the right profession for you. There are a number of different routes that you can take when it comes time to really narrow down your job search. Before you begin applying to various facilities or employers to find the CNA position that's right for you, consider what will be a match for your personality and career aspirations. Ask yourself some rather important questions as you begin your job search, such as:

- Do I plan to remain as a CNA or is this just a stop in my overall nursing career?

- Do I intend on focusing on patient care solely or wish to learn more that can lead me to future opportunities?
- Am I cut out to work in an emergency type of setting?
- Do I intend on having a specialty within my nursing career?
- Are there facilities that are close to my home that may work out in terms of convenience?
- Are there certain places that may pay more than others?
- Do I wish to work as a part of a team or will I do better working independently?
- Do I want to get a taste of various types of nursing care?
- Would I enjoy working on individualized patient care, perhaps even out of their home?
- Would I consider temporary or contract work as I get started?

There are so many questions to ask yourself to be sure that you get an accurate measure on what the right nursing assistant career is for you. As with the decision to become a nursing assistant, this too is a personal choice and everybody is going to have a varying view on it. Some people may enjoy strictly focused patient care because they feel that this is why they obtained their CNA and where they plan to stay with things. You have to ask yourself the tough questions and truly evaluate why you went into the nursing assistant profession and what your long term career goals really are. Only you can decide upon these aspects and every nursing assistant will take a different path, the right one is truly up to you.

Career Options

Most people outside of the nursing profession would never have an idea of just how many options lie before an individual who gains their CNA certification, but there opportunities are almost limitless. If you keep up with current events, you will quickly see that this is a hot profession right now. The need for nursing assistants is on the rise and shows no signs of slowing down anytime soon. This is great news for the people already in the profession and particularly for those just entering their career as a nursing assistant. This means that you have options, and this is a great distinction from so many other fields out there. As the need for qualified health care and excellent patient care continues to rise, so too does the need for certified nursing assistants who bring experience to the table. All great for an individual about to finish their CNA training!

This also means that you don't have to settle and that depending on your area of the country, that you just might have some excellent choices before you. In the past, you may have been "pigeonholed" into a job at a nursing home as that was the only facility with the needs for a nursing assistant, now you can find some truly "out of the box" opportunities as well as some excellent stepping stones in your nursing career. Think about what's important to you, what's going to teach you the most, and where you intend on ultimately ending up, and then plan your career around all of that. You can make this all work for yourself. So consider this, looking at all of your many options can help you to focus on what you truly want to do. A profession as a nursing assistant can entail a great deal of things and opportunities. Some possible opportunities for a CNA include the following:

- Working at a nursing home
- Working through a temporary nursing placement agency
- Working with individual patients who require their own private nursing assistant
- Doing home nursing care
- Working as a nursing assistant at a hospice facility to help keep patients happy in their terminal illness
- Working at a hospital
- Working at an outpatient medical facility assisting with patient care in the operating prep or recovery rooms
- Working at a health clinic
- Working at an urgent care facility that requires nursing assistant help
- Picking a specialty or focus and lining up a nursing assistant job that will help you to gain the necessary experience
- Working with bed ridden patients on helping with all of their needs through the appropriate medical facility

This is only the tip of the iceberg because if you start getting into certain specialties or specific areas of the country, you will be sure to find so many other wonderful opportunities out there. Don't limit yourself—think through what would really make you happy in your career as a nursing assistant and then focus your efforts on finding a job within that particular field. This is where it really pays to ask yourself the tough questions up front and ensure that you are going about your job search the right way.

Background Checks For Nursing Assistants

In today's society, background checks are conducted by most employers to help safeguard against theft as well as to help secure the safety of the people they serve and the other staff members. Anyone wanting to be a Nursing Assistant should expect a very thorough background check to be conducted prior to being hired at any medical facility. In many instances, a background check will have to be completed prior to acceptance in a Nursing Assistance program. It generally depends on the state requirements.

The level of clearance you must pass on a background check varies by agency and state. In some states, only crimes involving violence will ban you from employment as a Nursing Assistant. In others, any felony will result in not being hired. There are a few states that push it even further. If you have any history of domestic violence, harassment, drunk driving, misdemeanors, or felonies, you can't work in the medical profession.

While some may think this is extreme, statistics show theft and abuse committed by Nursing Assistants is done by those who have some criminal record prior to being hired by the agency where the abuse or theft took place.

If you are not familiar with a background check, it can include many things. Some employers simply check your criminal history. Others go to great lengths to find out information about you. They will check the education information on your resume, verify all past employment, and call all your references. There are a select few employers who will conduct a credit rating as well. This is because up to 40% of all resumes given to employers contain some kind of false information.

Investigating a person's motor vehicle record has also become popular. The one area that an employer can't look into is your medical history. However, many medical facilities require Nursing Assistants to pass a physical exam prior to hiring.

An employer will need to discuss the types of background checks they will conduct prior to doing so. Often, you will need to sign consent from allowing them to obtain such information. In most cases, an employer will not be conducting a background check unless they are ready to offer you the job. It is not uncommon for them to offer the position, but clarify that it is contingent on the background check coming back clear.

This being told, Nursing Assistants need to be up front about their background. While it is difficult to secure employment in the field with a criminal history, it is possible depending on the circumstances. If you lie about your work experience, it is quite possible you will get caught. Since the demand is so high for Nursing Assistants, you can still get the job if you don't have much work experience. Employers are often looking for someone who is honest and willing to work. Show them both, and they will offer to train you.

If your background check comes back with information that negatively reflects your chances of being hired, the company has to provide you with the information they received as well as the name of the company they obtained the information from. If they information is incorrect, it is very important that you contact your local agency relating to the reported information. In addition, remember that getting into trouble with the law, the Department of Motor Vehicles, or financially might result in you losing your position as a Nursing Assistant. You will want to review the policies for the agency you are accepting employment with.

Job Search Guidelines

Though the fact that a nursing assistant is in high demand works to your favor, you still need to be prepared in order to successfully find the job of your dreams. Some areas of the country are easier than others to find a great job, and also have some excellent resources available. It's on you though to take the necessary steps required to land yourself a job that will make you truly happy as a nursing assistant. Even with the number of jobs available, that doesn't translate to the jobs falling into your lap. You have to put forth the work to find a great job, just as you put forth the work to find a great CNA program. As you studied your curriculum and observed in the training portion of your certification, the job search is a true process.

If you follow the required and recommended steps it will help you to find something that is truly a match for you and for which you can be happy with for a long time. Even if there are a great number of jobs out there for nursing assistants, it doesn't mean that the first one you find is the best match. Take your time, do your research, gain some perspective, focus on what's truly important to you, and begin the process towards finding the nursing assistant job that is an excellent match for you. So what are the steps in the job search process?

1. Prepare a Detailed Resume: Think of things that will make you stand out from the crowd. Be sure to list out any related or pertinent experience, what value you bring to the table, or what you can offer to help set you apart from other nursing assistants you may be competing against. If you think along these lines, you are sure to create a resume that will blow people away in the job search process.

2. Do Your Research: Take the time to research what options are available in your area and do this early on. Educating yourself is a huge part of the process and a surefire way to get to the successful career you are after. Being proactive is what will set you apart from the competition. Rather than just

waiting for a nursing assistant job to come your way that may or may not meet your goals and objectives, take the time to research what your options may be. There may be new needs popping up, new medical facilities opening up, or something that fits within your specialized or specific needs.

3. Write Down Your Goals and Aspirations: When your goals are tangible and visible, they become much more attainable. Decide upon what is important to you so that you can focus your job search efforts on it. If you want a longer term or more specialized career within the nursing world, then by all means document it. If you want to become well versed with patient care and become established at a given facility, then write that down as well. Having something to look forward to and work towards makes you better and this is especially important at the beginning of your nursing assistant career so you are clear on where you want to head. As your goals or objectives change, write them down and keep on top of them moving forward.

4. Network and Make Connections: Even though a CNA is a "hot" job that is in high demand right now, it can be extremely beneficial to make connections. Talk to people in your related field,

make connections with those that may be in a specialized field that you are ultimately interested in, and join any possible organizations in your area. You can even find online forums that can be of great help in the networking world to point you in the right direction for your goals. It takes one contact to get you to the nursing assistant job of your dreams, so talk to people that can help you to get there.

5. Make a List of Possible Avenues and Then Apply to Them: Whether they show a job opening or not, sometimes a proactive attempt at an application can open a door for you. After performing your research, make a list of the types of facilities that interest you and then determine where these exist in your area. Send a personalized cover letter, your resume, and an application or any other required documents to successfully apply for employment with that potential employer. If you find that the facilities you are interested in are not activity hiring, then try to gain access for an informational interview. Just do what you can to tactfully and successfully get your foot in the door and make the opportunity happen for yourself.

6. Interview Well: Even if there is not a job opening, simply setting up an informational interview or initial meeting is a proactive measure that can truly

pay off. You want potential employers to remember you for all the right reasons and have you come to mind when they envision the right person for their job opening. Rely on your experience and your personality to do well in an interview. Do whatever interview preparation you can such as studying up on the medical facility you are meeting with. Be prepared to answer questions about your background or situational based scenarios so that employers see how you would handle typical situations. Always put your best foot forward and a big part of that is being prepared and proactive so that the employer sees that you put forth all of the necessary effort to land the job.

7. Follow Up as Necessary: This is a step that a lot of people forget and it's an important one. Following up immediately after an interview, even if it's a proactive or informational one, can truly set you apart from the crowd. Thanking potential employers for their time and reiterating your interest just might be the necessary step required to help you land the job and get to the nursing assistant position that you are truly after. Remember that professionalism can go a long way and help you to achieve your career goals.

Finding the perfect nursing assistant position is a matter of being prepared. As you begin researching programs and find one that is a great fit for you, it is at this time that you should really ask yourself what you wish to accomplish with your CNA career. If you strive towards the true position that you want and focus your job finding efforts on it, you will land it. It may take time but it will lead you to the path that's right for you as a nursing assistant. This is important if you plan to stay where you land for awhile or even if you intend on moving onto a registered nurse profession. Thinking through what you really want out of your career and then actively going after it is what will lead to success as a nursing assistant.

The Pay Scale For Nursing Assistants

Nursing Assistants are a valuable part of our medical facility staff. They offer ongoing care to patients at level most other staff don't have the time to. They tend to basic needs of bathing, feeding, and dressing. They also provide emotional support to the patient and the family. Nursing Assistants are expected to help other medical staff at a moments notice with a variety of tasks including setting up medical equipment and getting patients ready to be taken for X-rays and surgery.

Most people entering the Nursing Assistant field don't do it for the pay. They do it out of a desire to be of assistance to others in need as well as a desire to work in the medical field. Since medical facilities rank Nursing Assistant as an entry level position, they pay is very low compared to others, especially nurses. This can lead to some Nursing Assistants feeling angry, upset, and unappreciated.

The median expected salary for a Nursing Assistant in the United States is $24,383. On average, that is approximately $2,000 per month. That amount varies by experience and job location. As you can see, it does pay more than minimum wage and often employees in this field are able to secure health insurance and retirement plans.

However, when you compare that to the median salary of a Licensed Practical Nurse, which is $43,333, you can see a huge different. While it is understood that the Licensed Practical Nurse position holds more responsibility and well as requires more schooling and training, we can also see why some Nursing Assistants feel that they aren't earning enough. It is also common that the better a Nursing Assistant is paid, the more pride they take in offering quality services to all patients.

Many health care facilities understand this, and work hard to keep Nursing Assistants content. They try to give raises as they can for performance as well as the length of time on the job. They understand that Nursing Assistants are vital to the overall balance of the Nursing staff. They also realize finding qualified employees is hard enough without having to continually interview and train new staff. Since Nursing Assistant jobs are plentiful, they can lose their good employees to other facilities who offer better pay.

Due to the pay difference, some individuals choose to go to school directly into a degree program and skip the Nursing Assistant certificate program all together. For those wanting to ease in the doorway of the medical profession and those who need the income while in school, the Nursing Assistant program is still very valuable to them in terms of having an income and being in a learning environment of the medical field.

The pay scale difference can often result in issues arising between Nursing Assistants and the Nursing staff. On one side, you have Nursing staff feeling that they have a degree and shouldn't have to participate in particular tasks. Others just are overwhelmed by time restraints, and therefore keep their job segregated from that of the Nursing Assistants. On the other side you have Nursing Assistants who feel their tasks are harder and they aren't getting paid nearly as much as the Nursing staff. This can lead to them developing feelings of resentment towards the Nursing staff. This being said, it is important for administration to help both the Nursing staff and Nursing Assistants interact and appreciate each other.

Seeing that pay difference as well as wanting to participate in more advances areas with the patients has lead many Nursing Assistants back into training to earn a degree as a Licensed Practice Nurse, a Registered Nurse, or another specified area in the medical field.

Medical facilities and the government agree that when medical staff is short, the patients are the ones who suffer the most. It is no different in the area of Nursing Assistant. If they positions aren't filled, the patients may not get all of their needs met daily. For example, some nursing homes only bathe the patients every other day because of short staff issues.

The government is trying to find funding to help increase the rate of pay for Nursing Assistants. However, they feel that they pay isn't the only issue. It is believed that healthcare facilities need to start showing Nursing Assistants more respect, appreciation, and recognition for their hard work. This profession has one of the highest turn over rates do to demanding work conditions, feelings of being under valued, and lower pay than most feel they are worth. The result is healthcare facility patients feeling the burden in part because of the pay scale for Nursing Assistants.

5

PRACTICE YOUR PROFESSION

You've finally done it! You've landed the job that you really wanted and are about to embark on your first days as a nursing assistant. It may have seemed like a long road, but if you are in a career that you truly love doing the things you really want to do it was worth it. Now it's time to settle back and enjoy what you do? Not really, it's time to keep sharp and constantly better yourself in your profession as a nursing assistant. This is the type of profession where sitting back on your laurels will never work. You are constantly thrown into new situations, asked to perform new tasks, or bettering yourself for the next step in your career. Even if you intend on staying as a CNA as your chosen career path, it's extremely important to stay sharp. Not only that, but to stay a Certified Nursing Assistant, it's a must to keep up on your continuing education credits so that you maintain your gained certification each and every year.

So you've worked hard, done all of the necessary research and preparation to land the job, and are ready to enjoy it. Now what? Now is the time to really utilize the certification that you worked so hard for and to practice it within your profession. Within a nursing assistant profession, there is always the opportunity to keep getting better and continuing to improve upon your skills and your performance. When it comes to patient care, you will likely be faced with new situations and adventures each and every day and week. You will likely learn new things as you continue on within your career, far beyond what you ever learned in your training in your CNA certification course. So how can you continue to improve? What can you do to practice within your profession and either progress to the next level or become one of the most trusted and best in your field?

Pointers For Developing Your Skills

It may seem that a career as a nursing assistant doesn't leave much room for perfection. Some may think that you are either good at patient care or are not, but that couldn't be further from the truth. While it may hold true that a career as a nursing assistant is a calling of sorts or that certain personalities are more well versed at it than others, the reality is that everybody can always improve upon their skills. There are some excellent ways to get started with sharpening your skills and some which may very well work throughout your career as a CNA. Whether a nursing assistant is the career of your dreams or simply a step towards becoming a registered nurse, there are ways that you can improve upon your performance and climb the ranks to be a trusted resource and one of the best in your profession.

After all of the hard work you've put into obtaining your CNA certification, it's time to put it to the test. This is where the best stand out from the crowd and where you can draw a line of distinction to show that you will in fact go on to be the best nursing assistant you can be. Here are some tips that will help you along your journey and allow you to truly practice what you've learned and keep getting better.

- If at all possible, find a mentor. While this is helpful in just about any profession, it can make for a huge distinction when it comes to moving on with your career or doing well where you're at. Let this person take you under their wing and teach you everything they know as this can help you to go from good to great very quickly.
- Ask a lot of questions. This sounds obvious but when some people are new to a profession, they are too shy to ask questions. If you want to get better and truly put what you've learned to the test, then you have to ask questions so that you know how to handle certain situations.
- Observe as much as you can. Even if there are situations that come up that aren't under your umbrella of responsibilities, take it all in. Observe what procedures are followed in certain situations or how you should react to patient care needs that come up. This will only help you to become a better CNA and ultimately get to where you want to be with your career.
- Talk to others in your field and compare experiences and techniques. This can be an excellent forum by which you can further your experience and get to the point you are happy with in your career. Understanding that people may do

things differently and that you can learn from others may help you to stay focused and work on your improvement.

- Never turn your back on potential experience. Each time you are presented with a new scenario, take advantage of it. Even if it seems like a rather unsavory or less than desirable job requirement, do your best to embrace it. Realize that as you practice all of these different aspects of your job responsibilities and progress through your career, each of these will prepare you as you move ahead.
- Study up as needed. If you find that you are struggling with various aspects of being a nursing assistant or that you require further development, go back to your education or find new sources to learn. To become more well versed and better at your career moving forward, you need to take the time to understand how certain things work. Educate yourself and recognize that as a nursing assistant, you are a constant work in progress.
- Enjoy what you do and work to always improve upon your job. You are responsible for continuing education credits, so be sure to focus your attention on areas that can make you better or for which you struggle within. At the same time, take the time to truly enjoy what you do and let it show. Even if you are only planning on being a CNA for a short while as you progress to other things, enjoy the job and learn from it, you may even make some great contacts along the way.

Continuing Education Makes You Stand Out

Though the tips surrounding how you can better yourself and truly practice your CNA certification within your profession may sound obvious, it's often ignored by many. Some may get into their job as a nursing profession and look at it as nothing more than that—just a job! While others may get into their nursing assistant role and really embrace it, but never figure out ways to better themselves or learn how to improve upon their performance. It's quite easy to become comfortable within your career or to think of it as just another aspect of your life. However as it takes a special personality to handle delicate patient care that lead you into the nursing assistant profession, it will also take the right attitude to progress. There are certain to be times that you will be challenged or feel that your career is not exactly what you envisioned, but try to embrace even those moments as opportunities.

Think back to what made you decide to become a nursing assistant and focus on it. After the long road of researching programs, getting into and excelling in a CNA certification course, and finding the job that was a good match for you, now it's time to really make it happen. This is a big step in your career and can set you apart from the rest of the pack if you open yourself up to the opportunities that lie ahead of you. Think about why you love what you do and what drew you to the nursing assistant profession and then apply that passion to the next major steps in your career. You are at an important and exciting threshold when you can practice what you've learned and figure out the ways to do it well.

With all the hard work that it takes to become a CNA, you should celebrate this new career as often as you can. Even when days get tough, you're doing something that you enjoy doing either as your final career destination or en route to an even broader nursing career. You've worked hard to find the job that you were after and now it's time to practice the skills that you've learned along the way. You will surely be met with challenges along the way, but you have arrived at your destination and now it's time to make it all work. It may have seemed intangible as you worked through the lessons in the classroom or practiced techniques in your on the job training, but this is it.

Being a nursing assistant is an excellent choice and there's a reason that it's a "hot" job right now—it takes a certain person to do the work that you are about to do so embrace it. You studied hard, practiced your skills, passed your test, went after the job you desired, and now it's time to make it all come together into a streamlined work flow. You've got what it takes so make it happen and allow all of your hard work, personality traits, and skills to come together to carve out a beautiful nursing assistant career path that's right for you. Going into the profession is an important decision and a huge commitment with a long path ahead of it, but once you arrive at the time to practice your skills and actually be a nursing assistant; this is what it's all about. This is the point at which greatness is made!

6

JOB SUPPORT

Being a Nursing Assistant is a very rewarding career for those who choose to enter the medical field with a thirst for knowledge and a dedication to helping others. Your Nursing Assistant course, clinicals, and trainings often don't prepare you for precautions you need to take. Most employers don't either. Therefore it is the responsibility of every Nursing Assistant to learn about them on their own.

Safety Precautions

One of the hardest parts of being a Nursing Assistant is taking direction from many other staff on the medical team. They are to report directly to the Nursing staff. It is not uncommon for each Nurse to have a slightly different way they want things to be done. This makes the job of the Nursing Assistant even more challenging. You need to be willing to stand up for yourself and the other Nursing Assistants.

If this type of issue is ongoing in the medical facility you work at, go to the charge Nurse. Explain why the changes among the Nursing staff are confusing and counter productive. Most charge Nurses will look into the situation, and help put policies, procedures, and trainings into place so that all staff knows exactly how something needs to be done.

Nursing Assistants are often required to life patients while bathing, dressing, or even getting them ready to go eat. It is important that you are properly trained in this procedure, or you can injury your back or other body parts. You also run the risk of causing injury to the patient. Since medical facilities are often short staffed, Nursing Assistants try to lift patients alone when they know they are to have a partner assist them. This is dangerous to your health, to your patient, and to your job security. Never cut corners on such practices no matter how much time they save you.

Communicable diseases are very important to avoid as a Nursing Assistance. You will likely be trained in communicable diseases both in your Nursing Assistant training and your employment orientation. However, it is important to remember that most communicable diseases are spread through bodily fluids. No matter how tight your time schedule is, if you find a patient has soiled their clothing or bed, make sure you use rubber gloves, clean the area properly including using a disinfectant, and wash your hands thoroughly with soap and water. This will help reduce you risk of infection from communicable diseases.

Many patients who require the care of a Nursing Assistant don't want it. This can lead to a variety of feelings including depression, being upset, anger, and hatred. Often, this mix of feelings gets released onto the Nursing Assistant. You may find yourself receiving verbal abuse and sometimes physical abuse from patients as a result. It is very important that you deal with this type of situation immediately. For verbal abuse, tell the patient you understand they are upset but that you are there to help them with… then proceed to tell them what you will be assisting with. Leave the room if they continue to be in that state of mind. Report the incident according to your employer's policies.

Physical abuse is more dangerous than emotional abuse. Patients need to understand that it will not be tolerated under any circumstances. If you have to defend yourself, yell for help or call out a code word according to your employer's policies. It is vital that you report any incident of physical abuse immediately to your supervisor. Document the incident including what took place, the type of physical abuse, and any self defense holds or moves you did to protect yourself. This becomes important if the patient later claims you abused them.

Avoiding burnout is another key area for Nursing Assistants to be aware of. This is the result of continually feeling overwhelmed by your job duties. The medical field ranks number one in the area of job burnout. It is important that you pay attention to burnout and these other precautions. This will enable you to further enjoy your employment as a Nursing Assistant.

Dealing With Communicable Diseases

Communicable diseases are those that can be transferred from one individual to another. These include the common cold, tuberculosis, the flu, and HIV, herpes, measles, chicken pox, lice, and strep throat. Are of these are highly contagious. For those who already have medical issues, their immune system has a hard time fighting off anything else, so they are very susceptible.

Communicable diseases spread by human waste including saliva, stools, urine, blood, and other bodily fluids. Airborne droplets from the nose and mouth are also a common transmitter.

Since communicable diseases often spread like wildfire if not properly contained, it is everyone's responsibility to do all they can to maintain their own health. Washing your hands often is a very good place to start. Most germs can't survive soap and water. Nursing Assistants are encouraged to wash their hands more than most people because they are in constant contact with other people.

As a Nurse Assistant, it is your responsibility to immediately notify your supervisor if you develop the symptoms of any communicable disease. They can then determine a course of action. It may be recommended that you don't come to work until the communicable disease has run its course. Depending on the disease, you might be able to continue working with a respirator to prevent passing it to anyone else. In some cases, it may need to be reported to the health department.

Some communicable diseases can be cured with antibiotics such as strep throat. Others including the common cold will have to run their course. You can do your part by remembering to wash your hands, taking your vitamins, being current on all immunizations, and getting an annual flu shot.

Learning about these types of diseases is an important part of the Nursing Assistant program. Most medical facilities train all new employees in the area of communicable diseases. There is also ongoing training. While preventing the spread of communicable diseases is important in any work environment, it is especially important in a medical setting.

Each medical agency will have different processes and procedures for handling the spread of communicable diseases. Make sure you are well trained in identifying them, noticing the onset, and knowing how to handle each type of situation. Epidemics of communicable diseases require emergency procedures to take place. It is very important that you agency trains all employees in that area as well.

Nursing Assistances come into contact with bodily fluids of patients on a regular basis, and this is the most common method that they are infected with communicable diseases. You should always use rubber gloves when doing tasks such as changing soiled bedding and clothing and empting bedpans. The use of a sterile disinfectant while cleaning is important as well. If you do get bodily fluids on you, immediately was the area with soap and water, then report the incident. Your report needs to include what took place and what bodily fluids you came into contact with.

Communicable diseases are an area many people don't know much about. It is important that Nursing Assistants do some research on their own to make sure they fully understand the health risks involved with coming into contact with communicable diseases. While it is very rare, there have been reports of Nursing Assistants being infected with HIV and other potentially deadly diseases.

Dealing With Burnout

Those who decide to pursue a career in the medical field as a Nursing Assistant set out to show compassion and help others. Their hearts are in the right place, but they may soon find their minds and bodies suffering from burnout. This is the result of continually feeling like you can't meet your work requirements. Soon you find you are completely drained and exhausted due to feeling overwhelmed. Often, the result is losing the motivation that lead you to take on that role in the first place.

The role of a Nursing Assistant is a demanding one. One of the biggest complaints from them is that they have too much to do, and not enough time to get it all done. Burnout is dangerous because it affects individuals emotionally, physically, and mentally. It is tough to see bright, compassionate Nursing Assistants leave the medical field because they have come to resent the role they have taken on. It no longer serves a purpose for them.

What was once a positive experience has become a nightmare.

The stress of burnout on a Nursing Assistant can lead to problems with their health as well as lead to depression. Often, they either quit their job or they are fired. This leads to financial difficulties and many times issues in their relationships. Nursing Assistants report burnout in their profession is common because they are overworked, unappreciated, confused about work expectations and priorities, worry about job security, they are overwhelmed by the number of responsibilities, and they do not feel their pay is sufficient for the amount of duties that they are required to perform on an ongoing basis.

It is important that Nursing Assistants understand burnout, and the havoc it can reap in their professional and personal life. Understanding what burnout is, why it happens, and the signs of it can help Nursing Assistants deal with the situation before it spirals out of control. The first step in avoiding burnout is to take care of yourself physically and emotionally.

Signs you are experiencing job burnout or soon will be include no longer finding enjoyment in areas of your job you once really liked, becoming cynical or bitter about your job, and you are starting to experience problems in relationships with co-workers, friends or family as a result of the conflicts of your job.

Other important signs to watch for are looking for excuses to not go to work, calling off or asking to go home early on a regular basis, becoming easily annoyed with co-workers, envious of those who do enjoy their work, and not caring if you do a good job or not. It is likely you will start to experience physical and emotional exhaustion.

Being a Nursing Assistant can be stressful. However, stress and burnout are different. They are often confused because they signs and symptoms of the two are very similar. The defining factor is stress comes and goes, so the signs and symptoms do as well. With burnout, the feeling doesn't go away, so the signs and symptoms linger ongoing.

As a Nursing Assistant, you can't eliminate stress, but you can help control and reduce the effects of it. It is important to get plenty of rest and take care of yourself. Since most of us stretch ourselves too thin with too many commitments, see if there are areas you can cut back in. If you have solutions to issues at work, write them down. Ask to meet with your supervisor. Explain the problems, then offer solutions. This will show that you are interested in resolving the issues rather than just complaining.

It is very important to take time for yourself. Relax with a warm bath or read a good book. Too often we take care of everyone else's needs at work and at home, leaving nothing of ourselves for us! Since the healthcare profession is the top contender for employees suffering from burnout, Nursing Assistants need to really take head of this advice and put it to good use early on in their career. This will help ensure they continue to enjoy their work, offering patients the best possible care.

Counseling For Nursing Assistants

The day to day activities of a Nursing Assistant can be rewarding and draining. Most of us only know that they offer assistance with feeding, dressing, and bathing patients. However, they do so much more. They develop ongoing relationships with the patients as they have more one on one time with them than any other medical staff. They also provide comfort to the patient and their family. They do all they can from reading to them, helping them write letters, and holding their hand as they move from life to death.

Experiencing the negative activities that occur in the Nursing Assistant profession can really take a toll on an individual. It is especially hard when someone they have been caring for takes a turn for the work, becomes terminally ill, or dies. They still have to go on with their other patients, but they can be left feeling empty and at a loss.

Many medical facilities are aware of this issue. With being compassionate comes true feelings of friendship and loss. Counseling is a good way to help Nursing Assistants deal with the events that take place in the working environment. This counseling can be conducted through the employer or at the expense of the Nursing Assistant from an outside resource.

Counseling services offered on site to Nursing Assistants is generally offered free of charge, as long as the information being discussed is work related. The employer may have several paid counselors that only provide services to employees. Others use their counselors to provide services to their employees, patients, and the family and friends of patients. You will need to look into how it is set up at your place of employment for specific details.

These counseling sessions can be ongoing or set up only when a Nursing Assistant feels the need to do so. It is important to understand that the information you discuss with the counselor at your worksite will not be shared with your employer. Too often, Nursing Assistants avoid this type of support and help because they are afraid their boss is going to get a transcript of the entire session. All counseling sessions are held in strict confidentiality. They only time anything is reported is if the counselor feels you are in danger of hurting yourself or others.

Since counseling is important in the medical profession, you may be able to encourage administration at your place of employment to set up services for employees. While they may argue that it is costly and not in the budget, be prepared to discuss the benefits to the overall effectiveness of the staff. Employees with good mental health will do a better job. They will also choose to continue employment longer than staff that needs counseling but does not receive it.

If your employer does not offer counseling services, it is important that you look into an outside resource for such services. The Nursing Assistant field can be draining and emotional. A key to staying on top of the game is to take care of yourself. This means both on a physical and emotional level. In reality, you aren't going to be effectively caring for patients if you haven't been taking care of your own needs. Counseling services can be expensive, but most health insurance plans cover them. If yours doesn't or you don't have health insurance, check in your area for discount programs and sliding scale fees.

Counseling services for Nursing Assistants is a vital key to staying compassionate and interested in your work. If you let the dark side of the profession consume you, then you will no longer be contributing to the well being of the patients you care for. Being a Nursing Assistant is a great opportunity to care for others and give something of yourself to society. However, it can't be stressed enough that you must take the opportunity and time to properly meet your own needs. This is one of the biggest reasons so many people in the medical field suffer from burnout. They simply do not take their own needs into consideration at the level they should.

Helping Nursing Assistants Cope With Dying And Death

Nursing Assistants are a unique group of individuals who are dedicated to providing patients with the best possible care. They work hard to make sure their basic needs are met. They often go the extra mile to provide patients and their families comfort. They are trained to work hard, multi-task, and assist Nurses with any type of emergency that arises on any given day. However, their goal is to help others feel better. Dealing with the harsh reality of dying and death can be very difficult for Nursing Assistants to deal with, especially for those new to the profession.

Dealing with the issue of dying and death is relevant in any field of the medical profession. It is even more common if you are working in a critical care of elderly care facility. This issue should be taken into careful consideration before a Nursing Assistant accepts a position in such a facility.

Since all people view death differently, a Nursing Assistant will be exposed to many things going on during this time, both with the patient and with their family members. For those who are very religious, praying and possibly figures from their Church will be present. Others are afraid to die, and fight for every last breath trying to hold on. Respecting the wishes of the patient and the family is very important during dying and death.

There are those Nursing Assistants who are upset when they have to deal with dying and death. They feel this is not what they signed up for. They want to help people. However, Nursing Assistants can be a great source of comfort and compassion for patients and their families during those precious last hours. Do all you can to keep the patient comfortable. Often, their mouths become very dry. Even if they don't appear coherent, attempt to give them ongoing sips of water or ice chips. The lips may begin to crack, apply Chap Stick or Vaseline to prevent soreness.

Caring for dying patients requires you to remember details about them before they became so ill. For example, if a patient asked to be turned often because of soreness, continue to rotate how they are laying. Pay attention to their body temperature and adjust bedding, air conditioning, and heating as needed. A person will often become cold in the hours before death, so it is important to keep them as comfortable as possible.

Some signs of death Nursing Assistants should be familiar with include the loss of muscle tone, the slowing of circulation, changes in breathing, and blurred vision. It is important that the Nursing Assistant document such changes in the patient's chart and immediately notify the charge Nurse of the situation.

While a patient is dying, the Nursing Assistant can help make the process easier for the patient. Adequate pain medications should be administered as needed to reduce the pain. Play the music the patient enjoys. Consider reading them a favorite book or Bible passages. Sometimes they will need extra comfort including someone to hold their hand. A Nursing Assistant can assume this role. Often, Nursing Assistants can rely on each other to help make the situation easier. Many employers also offer counseling services if you feel they are necessary after dealing with dying and death of one of your patients. It is often easy to become attached to patients you care for on a regular basis. Your employer is well aware of this, and will want to help you feel better in your role as a Nursing Assistant.

Patient Rights Nursing Assistants Need To Be Aware Of

Nursing assistants take great care in providing patients with the best possible care. They assist with meeting their basic needs on whatever level that particular patient needs. Nursing assistants often have to make informed decisions for the patients they care for. However, it is very important for all Nursing Assistants to be aware of rights of all patients. Nursing assistants need to familiarize themselves with these rights and respect them.

Patients have the right to be fully informed at the time of admission and throughout their stay in the facility. As the Nursing Assistant, you may be asked questions by patients that you are not qualified to answer. Acknowledge this with the patient, let them know who can answer their question, and document the information in their chart. Most information given to patients and their family will come directly from the doctor or the charge Nurse.

All patients have the right to refuse treatment. This can be difficult for Nursing Assistants as they really want to be as helpful to the patient as possible. However, if they do not want your assistance you can't force them. You must report this to your supervisor as well as document the information in the patient's chart.

If a patient is not happy with the care they are receiving, they have the right to inquire about grievance procedures and file a complaint. If a patient voices a complaint to you, provide them with the information to file a formal complaint. The policies and procedures for doing so will vary be medical facility.

Patients shall not encounter physical or mental abuse from anyone while staying in a medical facility. This includes chemical and physical restraints. Any such incidents shall be reported by the Nursing Assistant immediately to the supervisor, and often the local police department.

It is the duty of all Nursing Assistants to provide each patient with confidentiality and dignity. They should be treated with respect and privacy in regards to their personal information. Keeping anything you find out in the medical setting confined to other professionals who must know the situation is the best advice.

Patients have the right to participate in the religion of their choice. They are allowed to have visitors from the Church as well as private visitors as long as it does not interfere with medical advice. The Nursing Assistant must learn to work the needs of the patient around such visits.

Providing quality care to individuals is a very rewarding challenge to Nursing Assistants. Keep in mind that each patient has their own personality, desires, and needs. They want these to continue being met even while they are in a medical facility. This allows them to maintain a routine and sense of normalcy. The longer you care for a patient, the better you will understand how to best care for them.

It is difficult to balance the medical needs of a patient with their own personal desires. However, it is possible to provide both by respecting the patient's rights. This will ensure that they understand and denied requests are done purely in the best interest of their well being. Nursing Assistants are often considered an ally by patients. They help reduce any issues between the patient and Nursing staff as well as the patient and physician.

Patient Abuse By Nursing Assistants

We have all heard horror stories of patient abuse by Nursing Assistants. This takes shape in many forms including sexual abuse, physical abuse, emotional abuse, and theft. Most medical facilities Nationwide are taking precautions against such abuse occurring, including completing background checks. In some states, you can't work as a Nursing Assistant if you have any charges relating to domestic violence, harassment, or drunk driving because it is possible such behaviors can escalate in the work environment.

Many organizations complain that Nursing Assistants aren't properly looked into because the demand is so great in the industry. As a result, some employers are lowering the background check expectations. However, many states are holding the employer responsible when such abuse occurs, so this will likely help to curb that process.

Sexual abuse charges by Nursing Assistants are taken very seriously. Such sexual abuse reports include allegations of inappropriate touching and sexual intercourse. It is most commonly found to take place with male Nursing Assistants with those they are responsible for bathing. It is the responsibility of Nurses to routinely make a surprise visit into the area where a Nursing Assistant is alone with a patient. This will help convey the message that their endeavors may be interrupted and caught.

Physical abuse by Nursing Assistants is often hard to prove unless it has been witnessed or bruises appear. Often this type of abuse is conducted by Nursing Assistants who are not satisfied with their job. They are easily upset, frustrated, and overwhelmed. Some abuse their patients as a method of teaching them that they think some of their behaviors are inappropriate. For example, some patients have reported being hit for soiling their clothes and bedding. This often goes unreported in elderly populations as they become very afraid.

Verbal abuse is one of the most common types of abuse by Nursing Assistants. It can be simple teasing, belittling, or threats. Often this type of behavior stems out of control issues and the desire to have a more important job.

Theft is the number one reported type of abuse by Nursing Assistants. In can include cash, food, jewelry, and even dietary supplements. In medical facilities, such theft can be hard to prove who did it because the patient comes into contact with so many individuals who work in the facility.

While most Nursing Assistants do their job with as much energy and work ethic as humanly possible, there are those who give the entire profession a bad name. It is sad when you think about it – when is the last time a Nursing Assistant who did a good job made National headlines? Yet let one fall out of line, and you will hear it on the TV, radio, and the internet continuously.

The Nursing Assistant profession can be very difficult. It takes a very particular type of individual to be able to meet the requirements. Employers have a responsibility to protect all the patients. This requires money and time to be spent on extensive background checks and training. It also requires workshops and ongoing training for all staff members. Everyone should know signs of abuse to be watching for and how to report them. Abuse by Nursing Assistants will be prosecuted by law. Anyone going into the profession needs to be made very aware of that.

Consumer Complaints About Nursing Assistants

Most Nursing Assistants work very hard to ensure the safety of patients as well as provide them with quality care. However, consumer complaints happen often, resulting in the profession not getting a fair look. Too often the focus is on the negative that takes place during interactions with Nursing Assistants than reporting good staff to the proper people.

One of the biggest complaints about Nursing Assistants by consumers is that they are too rushed. They often have to hurry through bathing and dressing because they have too many demands on their time in a given shift. This often results in patients getting cared for, but quickly and robotically. The personal touch is often smothered in an effort to get it all done.

For patients, simple requests are on of the few perks they have in a medical facility. It also allows they to still exercise some control over their decisions. This is very important to someone who no longer is able to be at home or do basic tasks for themselves without assistance. These requests can be as simple as helping them from the bed to a chair or bringing them a pen and paper to write a letter. It is easy for Nursing Assistants to get side tracked or forget. However, since these simply requests are important to the patient, it is very important that Nursing Assistants follow through with them. Carrying a pen and notepad to jot down requests is a great way to remember them.

Patients don't like to be kept waiting. It is very hard to adjust to. They may forget they are not the only patient. Nursing Assistants do the best they can to stay on schedule. However, working short staffed and medical emergencies can quickly put them behind schedule. Nursing Assistants have to prioritize, so sometimes helping someone who has fallen is more important than giving the patient a shower on time. Since confidentiality is so important, the Nursing Assistant can't tell the patient why they are running late.

Never discuss a patient with another staff member or family member in a manner that makes the patient feel as if they are not in the room. Speak with them in mind. It is important to carefully choose your words, even when you think they are asleep or in a coma. Many patients have filed complaints regarding conversations they overheard while Nursing Assistants thought they were sleeping or unresponsive.

One huge area of controversy is that many consumers are uneasy with who quickly a Nursing Assistant can obtain a license. They do not feel there is adequate training time to do an effective job. Federal guidelines require all Nursing Assistant programs to have a minimum of 75 hours of training. The actual amount will depend on the program coordinator and the state requirements for a particular program. However, it is often debated that to be certified as a manicurist, it takes over 1000 hours of training, but so little to become a Nursing Assistant.

Medical facilities and program developers defend the hours required to earn a certificate as a Nursing Assistant.

They feel the training builds on an individuals basic concepts of feeding, bathing, and dressing individuals. It is routine tasks we have all done at some point in our lives. They also stress that the clinical hours are hands on training in a medical facility with close observation. This type of training is more effective than just classroom curriculums of other programs. In addition, Nursing Assistants are closely supervised by Nursing staff on a regular basis.

Nursing Assistants work hard to do an effective job of meeting the needs of consumers. Complaints will continue to be file as long as Nursing Assistants maintain such high workloads. With the demand of this field continuing to grow, it is not likely that the workloads will get anything but larger over time.

Support Groups For Nursing Assistants

Working as a Nursing Assistant can be very fulfilling. It is a great feeling to know you spent your day helping others. However, with this job comes a great deal of stress and frustration at times. This is due to short staffing so there is too much to get done, issues with other medical staff, and dealing with terminally ill patients or those who have died while in your care. All of this can start to take a toll on a Nursing Assistant, both physically and mentally. As a result, many Nursing Assistants suffer from burnout. They no longer find joy in the profession they were once passionate about.

To help you manage the stress and other factors that your job as a Nursing Assistant brings, support groups are a great way to discuss how you are feeling, both the good and the bad. It is a way to create relationships and receive support from others in the same profession. You will also have the ability to provide support to others in the group.

There are many ways Nursing Assistants set up support groups. It is very easy to put up a flier at work and ask those who are interested to come to a meeting. Make sure your flier addresses the group is only for Nursing Assistants. Many employers will support this effort, and offer you a meeting place. Make sure you discuss your reasons for wanting to establish a support group to administration prior to advertising.

Some groups meet weekly while others meet every other week. You can have established topics for each meeting or just allow members to bring to the table what ever they want. Make sure to set up ground rules for respect as well as prevent the meetings from becoming nothing but complaint sessions. The purpose of the support group is to help you stay positive, not generate the negative.

If your group of co-workers is very small, you might decide to set up a Nursing Assistant support group in your community, inviting Nursing Assistants from all medical facilities to meet together. You can select a central location such as the library. Often Churches will allow groups to gather in their facilities when not in use. You can also choose to rotate the medical facility that will host each meeting.

Online support groups for Nursing Assistants have become very popular. They allow you a level on animosity that face to face meetings do not. Also, your group will consist of people from all over the Nation, not just in your area. This can lead to learning new ways that work well for others that you can apply to your work environment. Online support groups for Nursing Assistants are free to join. They also don't require an effort being put into reminders for meetings, or securing places to meet.

One such online support group called Nursing Assistant Central .com has thousands of members. They invite individuals thinking of entering the Nursing Assistant program, those who are in the program, recent certificate holders, and those employed as a Nursing Assistant. There are message boards and chat rooms to discuss hundreds of topics. There is even a section where individuals can post questions related to their job. This site offers support and relieve to individuals in the Nursing Assistant field everyday.

It is important for Nursing Assistants to be aware of the dangers of stress and burnout in their profession. Having a reliable support system in place is a great way to offset the effects of stress and burnout. While our families and friends are often supportive of our career choice, they don't understand the depth of some of the challenging issues that happen for Nursing Assistants in their job. Having a support group made up of your peers allows you a resource that is walking in the same shoes. If you are hesitant, give a meeting or two a try. You just might find it is exactly what you need to help you keep that level of enthusiasm for your job at its best.

Appreciating What Nursing Assistants Do

Nursing Assistants work very hard to offer a contribution to the medical field. They work hard to help patients meet their basic needs. They also offer comfort and support. They work one on one with patients, getting to know them better than the other medical staff. They use this knowledge to make things easier for the patient as well as to help the other staff do what is best for the patient. In addition, they work with Nursing staff, often assisting with anything that comes up at a moments notice.

While most Nursing Assistants are happy in their role, they often do feel like they are taken for granted. The do so much behind the scenes that often the patients and the employer don't realize all that they contribute to the overall goals of the medical facility and the medical profession as a whole. There are several things patients, staff, and employers can do to recognize the efforts of Nursing Assistants.

Many patients and their family choose to send a simply thank you note or letter to the Nursing Assistant. Often, this heartfelt thank you is more than sufficient. It can often help a Nursing Assistant stay motivated, knowing what they do really does make a difference for many people. A simple gift of candy, flowers, or a gift card can also be a great token of appreciation for someone who offered so much during your time of need.

Many Nursing Assistants do not feel appreciated by other medical staff, especially the Nursing staff they work directly under. Too often Nursing staff only point of what a Nursing Assistant didn't do. This needs to be addressed, and verbal appreciation needs to be expressed towards the efforts of Nursing Assistants. Another great way to show appreciation is to ask Nursing Assistants for their input regarding patient care and include them in discussions about how to handle particular patient issues. This will definitely make them feel appreciated and valued.

Employers need to work hard to make Nursing Assistants feel appreciated as well. With them being is such high demand, they need to work hard to keep those quality workers they already have. In addition, their attitude towards the issue will often set the tone for other medical staff.

Employers can extend appreciation to individual Nursing Assistants or the profession as a whole in employment newsletters. These are often well read materials that pertain to the medical facility and can be distributed monthly or every pay day along with your check. If your facility participates in Medical Appreciate Week, then it is imperative that the Nursing Assistants feel honored during that time as well. Some employers offer raises to Nursing Assistants based on their performance as a bonus to recognize their efforts.

It is important to understand that Nursing Assistants don't enter the profession looking for recognition. They sincerely want to help others the best way they can. However, being over worked and under appreciated it a mix that leads to stress, burnout, and often leaving the profession. Medical facilities need to take the opportunity to inform other staff of all the duties Nursing Assistants perform. Other staff and the facility need to work hard to make them feel as important as any other staff member. Too often, the mentality is that they are entry level workers with less education. This misconception will lead to a continued shortage of Nursing Assistants to help patients and other staff. That being said, it is definitely to the advantage of the staff and facility to make sure Nursing Assistants feel welcome, appreciated, and an intricate part of the team.

CONCLUSION

A career within the medical field at all is certainly not for everyone. There are a lot of less than desirable tasks that an individual must perform in any sort of medical role. To some this can be a turn off and therefore deter any interest and turn them away from any sort of related career aspiration. However for others, a career within the medical field is a true calling that reaches out to them, even as kids to certain individuals. If you are simply meant to be in the medical field, you know it and you feel it. That's what you hear so many people say, and that holds especially true for nursing assistants. To be a nursing assistant means to have a true love for patient care and a desire to handle whatever they may need. Sure it's not often glamorous, but to many this is the core of patient care and what so many go into the profession for. It's what makes the medical field great to be able to handle a patient's every need.

It matters not if you intend to go into the nursing assistant role simply as a stepping stone towards becoming a registered nurse or if it's your lifelong aspiration, either way it's hard work. This hard work is also one of the best teaching type of roles some would say because you are thrown into the trenches of patient care and handling needs that require patience, dignity, and a certain personality to be able to make the patient comfortable and happy. Many of the patients that you will deal with along the way have special needs or are in a bad spot in their life, and so you as a nursing assistant bring them the things that they can't do for themselves. This is what drives so many to become a Certified Nursing Assistant (CNA) and what keeps them motivated throughout their career.

It can be a long path at times along the way. Sometimes you can feel as though you are never going to reach the end or attain that dream job, but it will come with hard work and an internal motivation. Not everybody will follow the same path, but in summary here are the steps that individuals wishing to become a nursing assistant often follow:

- Make the Decision. Whether it's a calling or some research that has brought you to the platform of becoming a CNA, it's a big decision. Whether you've know that this is what you wanted to do your whole life or simply just came upon this career choice, make the decision that this is the direction you want to head and then stick with it. Be confident with your decision as this is an excellent career with great opportunities.
- Understand the Roles and Responsibilities of a CNA. There are a lot of misconceptions surrounding the role of a nursing assistant. There are many responsibilities that you will handle and then those that are designated for a registered nurse. As you have made your decision to become a nursing assistant, be sure that you understand what you will be focused on and what sort of work you will be doing when you find the right opportunity. There are some responsibilities that may be more difficult than others, but it can be a very rewarding career overall.

- Research CNA Programs. You have to consider your own lifestyle, schedule, limitations, and desires as you look for a CNA program. You want to make this all work from the start and ensuring that you get into the right program that will set the perfect tone for you is extremely important. There are many different types of CNA programs out there, all of which can cater to different individuals and their hectic lifestyles. You can find classes at a community college, major university, through a medical facility, or even online. Be sure to give proper thought to your decision so that you are sure to go with what will work best for you and allow you to put your best foot forward. The education and training that you get will form the basis of your career so think it through.
- Get Your CNA Certification. Each state has different requirements for their own individual CNA certification, so be sure that you research what you will need to do in your own state. On average, most states require about 75 hours in the classroom and 12 with practical or on the job training. This may sound like a lot, but it's extremely beneficial as it will properly prepare you for your role as a nursing assistant. It's important to remember that you have to successfully pass the certification exam when all is said and done, and that you must keep up with your continuing education to keep your certification as the years go on.
- Research Companies Hiring Nursing Assistants. The great news for those going into the nursing

assistant profession right now is that this is a "hot" job. Even in tough economic times, hiring for nursing assistants is on the rise. This is wonderful for those just getting their certification and just goes to show that even when times get tough, there's always a need for good solid patient care. This should also serve as a platform by which individuals should take the time to look into the opportunities that are good for them and not settle. As you go through the process of becoming a nursing assistant, remember that you want to end up somewhere that will allow you to practice your skills and really build up your experience.

- Practice Your CNA Certification. After a long road, you can really get into the heart of why you decided to become a nursing assistant in the first place. Whether it was a true calling or just simply something that you are doing on your way to become a registered nurse. Whether you always envisioned yourself working as a nursing assistant or it came to you as you decided what you wanted to do with your life, this can be a very rewarding and at times challenging role. All the hard work finally pays off when you get to care for patients that appreciate everything you can for them.

Patient care is certainly not for everyone, but those who decide to become a nursing assistant can appreciate that there are some excellent rewards. There are challenges along the way and some days that may prove to be difficult, but giving back by caring for those who can't care for themselves can make it all worthwhile. Making the decision to become a nursing assistant is a great one and through a few well throughout steps, it can be tremendously successful for you and your career aspirations. Be sure to think everything through each step of the way and you will very well end up with a lifelong career that allows you to practice the patient care that so many are after. Being a nursing assistant is an excellent career path and if you follow the steps that we've outlined for you here, you will find that it can be a smooth and enjoyable transition to a career that is sure to give you great satisfaction for years to come.

Looking to get your hands on more great books?

Come visit us on the web and check out our giant collection of books covering all categories and topics. We have something for everyone!

http://www.kmspublishing.com